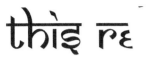 

this re ... gi

Everyday adv ... ga world

Daphne Kapsali

This Reluctant Yogi

Everyday adventures in the yoga world

First published by dk press in October 2015
Updated edition published in April 2017

Copyright © Daphne Kapsali, 2015

The moral right of the author has been asserted.

All rights reserved. No part of this publication may be
reproduced, stored in a retrieval system, or transmitted, in any
form or by any means, electronic, mechanical, photocopying,
recording or otherwise, without the prior permission of the
author.

"Switch off" published on Elephant Journal
Waylon H. Lewis C Enterprises 2014: Use Rights in perpetuity.
Ownership remains with author.

ISBN: 978-1545264614

For Polyna

This was supposed to be a post about 108 sun salutations, but it's been hijacked by my hamstrings. They are being, frankly, complete and utter bastards. I am far from impressed by the passive-aggressive attitude they've adopted towards me, and their muttered accusations – *recklessness, abuse* – are bordering on libel. They will not be pacified.

I have tried everything. I immersed them in scalding hot Epsom salt baths. I lovingly massaged them with essential oils. I rubbed magnesium oil, tiger balm and china gel into them. I gave them gentle stretches. I gave them rest. No good.

If they were a woman, I would buy them flowers and chocolate and deliver those items in some grand, romantic way (though not on my knees, as said hamstrings will not allow bending or squatting or any sort), along with a heartfelt note detailing all of my flaws, apologising profusely for my thoughtless behaviour, stating that I am truly not worthy and finally appealing to their kind and forgiving nature for redemption, and the ability to tie my own shoelaces again.

If they were my boyfriend, I'd cook them a delicious dinner, procure a few bottles of fancy Belgian beer, and then serve all of this up, along with myself, attired in my sluttiest outfit. I would praise them for their many manly attributes, and attempt to entice them with promises of all the acrobatic sexual feats I would perform – bendy yogi that I am – if only I could regain my ability to move my own limbs without whimpering.

Or I could write them an epic poem – *Oh hamstrings, ye art mighty* – and compare them favourably to other, lesser muscle groups. I could sing their praises like war heroes, acknowledging their selfless sacrifice for the greater good. They won't appreciate it, however. Though it pains me to admit it, my hamstrings are not all that cultured. And they're not heroes, either; they are martyrs. Because, I swear to you: they knew. We've all heard of muscle memory, but how about muscle precognition? I'm sure it's a thing. Those bastards knew, and they didn't say a word. They chose to martyr themselves in order to punish me.

May I get to it now? Thank you, hamstrings.

What I'm being punished for is this: 108 sun salutations against human trafficking. A pursuit I, perhaps misguidedly, joined at Triyoga Chelsea, one of hundreds of yoga studios around the world that took part in the annual Odanadi charity event on the 15th of March 2014. I somehow conceived of the notion that this would be a fun thing to do and, what's more, that I could do it. And, not satisfied with simply deciding that I'd do this in the privacy of my own head, where I could un-decide it at anytime without losing any yogi points, I announced it to all my colleagues and friends, and urged them, enthusiastically, to join me. Jill agreed. And, thus, my fate was sealed.

The hamstrings – may I point out – made no comment at

this stage.

And so I went about preparing for this task; I, a self-confessed reluctant yogi who laughs at the mere suggestion of taking a Vinyasa class. While Jill embarked upon 100 days of yoga, with numerous sun salutations thrown in for practice, and combined with walking to work – from Putney to Chelsea – on a regular basis, I, apparently, chose to focus on the mental aspect of my training, by meditating on the absolute impossibility of actually getting through 108 sun salutations and practising non-attachment to both this goal and my physical wellbeing. It was all very Zen. In fact, in the three weeks running up to the 15th of March, I did no yoga whatsoever, except to briefly demonstrate to my mum the difference between the sun salutation sequence I usually follow at home, and *Surya Namaskar A*, which was what was rumoured we'd be doing on the day. In addition to this, I ate an enormous amount of junk food (which I thoroughly enjoyed), followed by a four-day green smoothie cleanse, which left me feeling virtuous, lightheaded and ever so slightly deranged. And then the day of reckoning was upon me.

So there I found myself, bleary-eyed on a Saturday morning, with a beaming Jill next to me and a ticket in my hand, setting down my future like a fortune cookie:

108 SUN SALUTATIONS
07:15-08:15
STUDIO 2

Which is when Zen abandoned me and arithmetic kicked

in: 108 sun salutations. In an hour. ONE HUNDRED and EIGHT? In ONE HOUR? How is that even possible?

'Oh,' remarked a fellow yogi while we waited, lambs to the slaughter, for the session to begin, 'that's roughly two a minute'.

I looked around at the motley crew of brave, crazy people, all gathered here at 7 on a Saturday morning to salute a pale, London version of the sun one hundred and eight times, and expected them to bolt, one by one, for the exit. Nobody moved. They just nodded, happily and sagely, as if "two a minute" was somehow both achievable and a reassuring prospect.

And I thought: You are all batshit fucking crazy.

And: I am going to die.

Hamstrings: speak now or forever hold your peace.

Not a peep.

Enter Julie Montagu, our teacher, and – I have to admit – a source of apprehension for me on this occasion. Though I love Julie, I wasn't sure that her trademark upbeat teaching style would be what I needed to get me through this particular feat. This was a solemn pursuit, I reckoned, and should thus be undertaken with a degree of solemnity; I was resigned to laying my life down on my yoga mat For The Children, but I wasn't prepared to be cheerful about it. I was wrong: Julie was fantastic. After assuring me I wasn't going to die, she announced that, since we were all superheroes for being there, we would do our practice to a soundtrack of theme songs from superhero movies. She kicked us off with "Eye of the Tiger", which launched us on our journey in fits of giggles, and then led us through one hundred an eight repetitions of *Surya Namaskar A* (the rumours were correct), giving us the count at exactly the right points, so our spirits didn't wither and die. Counting us up one-two-three-four-five would have probably seen most of us give up before the halfway point, but the way Julie did it, we were up to 25 before we knew it. And so, to the tune of Batman, Superman, Spiderman, X-Men and Captain America, with a bit of Star Wars thrown in, we stretched up and dove down and looked ahead and jumped back and lowered down and pushed through and rolled back and jumped forward and folded down and flew up, and if you want it in Sanskrit, that's

Tadasana
Urdhva Hastasana
Uttanasana
Ardha Uttanasana
Kumbhakasana
Chaturanga Dandasana
Urdhva Mukha Svanasana
Adho Mukha Svanasana
Ardha Uttanasana
Uttanasana
Urdhva Hastasana

one hundred and eight times. And, in case you wondered: one hundred and eight is the precise number of Lord Krishna's most favourite consorts. (That's not the total number, you understand – only the favourites. Other, lesser consorts are not accounted for. Which is a bit ironic, given that, as I've been reliably informed, the Hare Krishnas are forbidden from engaging in sexual activity except for procreation. One can only conclude they must procreate a lot.)

So there you have it: one promiscuous deity, one hundred and eight consorts, a bunch of superheroes, and a set of hamstrings on their way to martyrdom. Because my wrists had started complaining even before Julie called out twenty five. Halfway through Krishna's lady friends, my shoulders were on fire, my biceps and triceps were screaming, my calves were in spasm and both my feet had cramped at least twice. Seventy five to ninety was the lowest point: my knees had turned to jelly, my abs were in turmoil, and there were sharp twinges of pain in my lower back as I staggered into plank and dragged myself forward into *ardha uttanasana*. My arms literally gave up, several times and without warning, and I collapsed on my face, in some grotesque parody of *chaturanga*, in a puddle of my own sweat, only to peel myself off and collapse again, on the way back to downward dog. But throughout all this, my hamstrings never said a word. Not a sound. Not even a polite cough or a gentle nudge. Absolutely nothing.

And so we made it to ninety and though I can't say I could see the light at the end of the tunnel, I at least became aware that there *was* a tunnel and an end to it and light. At this stage, to be entirely honest, I could hardly see anything through the sweat pouring down my face, and Julie's voice came from somewhere very far away, and I was vaguely aware of music but it was mostly drowned out by the gasping sounds that, presumably, came from me. And then Julie called one hundred and there was another, tiny, tentative voice whispering *you might actually get though this* and I did some stuff with my body and I breathed in and I breathed out and I remember thinking *I need to do these last ones properly* and

10

attempting to jump back into plank *mindfully*, using my core, or some such crazy nonsense, and then Julie said *that's it guys, that's a hundred and eight* and I collapsed into a sticky, sweaty heap of twitching limbs, next to a remarkably composed, rosy-cheeked Jill, before surrendering to the most well-deserved *savasana* ever.

And then, eventually, Jill and I made our way to the Chelsea Quarter café, where we had eggs royale and coffee and said very little, because our minds were still trying to come to terms with what we'd just done, and the effort of lifting our forks to our mouths was almost all-consuming, and slowly whichever spell we had been under that turned us, briefly, into superheroes began to disperse, leaving us with nothing more than a Saturday afternoon, a strange, disembodied sensation, and the urge to assert that we were "just a man and his will to survive". And three lessons:

1) Songs are written for superheroes, not martyrs. The most martyrs might hope to get is a hymn, or a prayer along the lines of *Oh hamstrings, show unto me mercy*, whereas dudes like Batman, shady character though he is, get cool capes and masks and gadgets and theme tunes, and even Rocky, arguably not a hero at all, gets "Eye of the Tiger". Which – no matter what your feelings on it might be – you cannot get out of your head.

2) There is no occasion solemn enough that it can't make you laugh.

3) Krishna must have been exhausted: one hundred and eight is a hell of a lot of consorts.

(If you want to know how my hamstrings are doing, you'll have to ask them yourselves; they're not talking to me.

Like those women who, after insisting they are *fine*, refuse to sleep with you for a week because *you don't even know what you've done*, my hamstrings have been blanking me for days now. I am not giving in; I was a superhero once, and I will not be bullied by any set of muscles.)

switch off

Having completed his early morning ritual of meditation, asana and pranayama, Swami Somethingorother is ready to draw his practice to a close. The sun, which has risen over the mountaintops, casting its dusty light across the ashram, has been saluted several times, and he has enacted various warriors, cats, dogs, and cows, as well as a number of undomesticated animals. His heart has opened up like a lotus flower, and he has attained a state of almost bliss, which he will now seal into his consciousness by means of a closing meditation and long, deep savasana. As he lays himself down on his yoga mat, he becomes aware of a gentle vibration in the vicinity of his right shoulder. Rolling himself over in its direction, Swami Somethingorother hoists himself up mindfully and reaches for his iphone: a text from Guru Important Dude, reminding him to mind his bandhas. He lays himself down again, adopting the Most Sacred Mobile Device mudra (where the thumb is deployed on the keypad and the fingers gently cradle the device, in a supportive manner), and fires off a reply to Guru, expressing his most profound gratitude. Being a practical man, he then quickly checks his facebook page for new likes (five), and skims his twitter feed for status updates from the other monks regarding their progress along the path to enlightenment. He notices he has three new emails, but decides to tackle those after his karma yoga practice, and before satsang. Satisfied, he places his phone back down beside him, arranging his physical body into savasana, and drifts into his chidakasha, that space of inner consciousness, breathing in and breathing out, as he brings his attention to his sankalpa: I am a kind and humble yogi, with a huge following on twitter.

What is wrong with this picture?

If your answer is *nothing*, or that Swami really ought to be focusing on his Instagram presence rather than twitter, you are beyond help, and I will ask you to kindly put this book away right now, and go take a selfie in headstand or something.

If, however, you are somewhat discomfited by the presence of Swami's mobile phone, if you're thinking that it doesn't quite belong in this context, then perhaps we have something to talk about. And it's all about *context*. If Swami really should know better than to use his mobile phone in the ashram, why would you take yours to class? Because you do; so many of you do.

I'm not perfect. I'm very much attached to my iPhone, to the point where I truly can't imagine life without it. But after two years of working in a yoga centre that proclaims itself a mobile-free zone, my phone spends most of its time on silent, forgotten in a coat pocket or buried in my bag. And I like it that way. After two years of being the mobile phone police, gently reminding people, several times a day, to please not use their phones in the centre, and being told, more often than you'd think, that it's just one phonecall, that it's urgent, or, quite simply, to fuck off (my lovely, very polite colleague was actually shown the middle finger *mudra* on one such occasion), I have become acutely aware of both context – a time and a place – and the sense of propriety and impropriety that's attached to it. I often find myself wanting to remind people that they cannot use their phone on the bus, but they can and I don't. And although context can sometimes be an abstract concept, there is nothing abstract about a yoga studio. If there is a time and a place for everything, mobile phones clearly do not belong in a yoga class.

And yet you see it every day. New converts or long-time yogis, wholeheartedly and earnestly embracing the yoga practice that has changed their lives, arriving early or late or just on time for the class that they absolutely cannot miss, and going into the studio armed with their class ticket, their bottle of water and their mobile phone. You see it in the studio, in that beautiful geometric arrangement of human bodies on yoga mats in neat rows along the clean white floor, and the harmony violently broken up by those dark rectangular intruders, placed at arm's length between the mats, literally or metaphorically vibrating with pent-up messages. You see it when these same people, who chant *om* and bring their hands into prayer and bow their heads and whisper *Namaste*, reach for their phones *the second* the class is officially over.

Context: let's broaden it a little bit. Yoga is much bigger than a class; it's so much more than the *asanas* you practice. It's actually this huge, ancient thing that none of us fully understand, and we have Westernised it and packed it up tightly and put it in a shiny package to make it more accessible and less terrifying. And that's fine, because we don't live in an ashram, and there is no space for the full ancient hugeness of yoga in our little Western lives. But we still need to remember what it is and where it came from, and that being part of it is a privilege. We are guests here, travellers at best, tourists at worst, and this place we're visiting has its own set of rules. And, as guests, the least we can do is respect them. And leave our gadgets at the door.

Louise (my most favourite teacher, and an excellent choice for reluctant yogis) never lets her students get away with bringing mobiles into class. 'You don't *necessarily* need your phone right now,' she says, kindly but sternly, and then she makes a joke about perhaps being old fashioned. But yoga *is* old fashioned. Don't be fooled by the shiny packaging, the glossy flyers or the state-of-the-art studios. Yoga is not some cool new thing we invented to make ourselves sound interesting and spiritual while toning our abs in preparation for the summer holidays; it isn't an intellectual version of bums 'n' tums or an alternative to spin. And even describing it as a lifestyle choice doesn't quite do it justice, somehow: lifestyle is a modern concept, and yoga predates it by thousands of years. Yoga is a way of living, which means, to put it very crudely, that you've got to take it in, and take it on, and take it outside the studio. Because it doesn't matter how many sun salutations you do each morning before breakfast. It doesn't matter if you've mastered the Ashtanga Third Series, or if you can scratch the back of your neck with your toes whilst balanced on one hand. It doesn't matter if you meditate on your lunch break. If you check your messages during class, you're not practising yoga. If you stroll out of the studio and leave your mat and props on the floor for someone else to put away, you're not practising yoga. If you walk out onto the street after class and flip out on the traffic warden issuing you a ticket because you parked illegally, you're not practising yoga. Take it on. Take it in. Take your yoga with you wherever you go.

But let's start small, and narrow it back down again: one class. On average, 75 minutes of your day. Leave your phone out of it. Like Louise once pointed out, *if you can't put your phone away for an hour and fifteen minutes, you shouldn't be in class at all.* You might as well take yourself back to the gym, where you can check your email while running on the treadmill, monitor your heart rate and update your Instagram account with sweaty, red-faced selfies, all at the same time. And take Swami with you; I have a feeling he'd really enjoy a spin class.

moontalk

On the night of the April full moon, Susanne and I spoke on Skype.

'I've just come back from my friend's place,' she said. 'We did a full moon ritual.'

'A *what?*'

A full moon ritual, she repeated. Whereby you hold a clear quartz crystal up to the full moon, and tell it what you want from life.

'And the moon will grant it?'

Susanne confirmed it would.

'OK,' I said. 'I have a quartz crystal, as it happens. I think I'll have a chat with the moon.'

'Do it,' Susanne urged, 'but be very specific.' That age-old warning: *be careful what you wish for.* Like magic lamps, moonlight and quartz crystals may come at a price. And if there is such a thing as a free lunch, it might not be exactly what you ordered.

Forewarned but undeterred, I said goodnight to Susanne, fetched my crystal from my desk (quartz crystals are said to protect against radiation, so mine lives by my computer screen) and drew aside the curtains of my single, tiny window over Battersea Park Road. As luck would have it, the moon was right there: round and huge and bright, shining down on South West London on a rare, cloudless night. Taking this as an auspicious sign, I climbed up on my bed to open the window, and pushed my hands – and the crystal – through the narrow gap and over the busy street below. The wail of police sirens, the roar of bus engines and a bass-heavy hip-hop tune from a car stopped at the traffic lights on the corner came rushing into my room, but I fixed my faze on the moon and focused. I didn't have to think for long: I know what I want and it *is* very specific. There was a moment of uncertainty when I realised I knew nothing about this ritual except that it involved a crystal and the moon. But something told me the crystal should be held in both hands, and that *Namaste* – palms together – should come into it at some stage. So I held the crystal up to the moon until I got the angle right and the moonlight shone through and then, having established a connection, I pressed it between my palms, with arms outstretched, and I talked to the moon in my head, and I told it what I wanted.

I said some good and true things, and I thought about the moonlight and my crystal and myself, and how the three of us were linked, in this moment, and about the whole universe of potential and possibility that contained all the things I wanted and which were connected to me and the crystal and the moon in exactly the same way, and I called them to me. And then I touched the crystal to my forehead and my heart, and gazed up at the moon until my eyes stung and watered, and then I bowed my head, said 'thank you', and shut and window and jumped off the bed, and the ritual was over.

And I would have thought no more about it, or perhaps mentioned it anecdotally, in passing, if it weren't for the fact that a few days later a man appeared on my doorstep, and he was exactly what I'd asked for. And just to clarify: I didn't actually ask for a man, and I didn't ask for this man, in particular, though he has been in my life for many years. If all I wanted was a boyfriend, I'd join Tinder; I'm sure the moon has better things to do than to play matchmaker to randy Londoners. Nor is it in the habit of delivering flat pack boyfriends to your door, like some cosmic IKEA. What I asked for is much bigger than that, and it doesn't come with instructions for putting it together: joy and fulfilment on a professional, intellectual, emotional, creative and spiritual level; kindness and love and peace, for myself and those around me. Just like my crystal, I have many facets, and I've gotta get the angle right, and expose them all to the metaphorical moonlight, if I am to function as a whole. I may be new to this, but I intuitively understand you shouldn't focus on the means but on the end, and trust whichever forces are at play to provide the means they deem most appropriate, even though they might surprise you. And the end, for me, is as simple and as complicated as this: to be myself, the best and truest version of all that I can be. And then, next to me, side by side, a person who accepts me exactly as I am. Not someone to fill a gap, but to stand beside me; two wholes that happen to fit together, and drive each other forward, in a journey that's both separate and joint. I explained all this to the moon, and it gave a nod. 'Alright,' it said.

Before you start rolling your eyes, before you dismiss me as some crazy new age fool, I will ask you to suspend your judgement for a moment longer, and bear with me while I try to explain: I have spent the last two years working in a yoga studio. Immersed in a world where talking about chakras and referring clients to a medicine man who does egg readings is as routine as checking the inbox for email enquiries (which, incidentally, were often headed "*Sat Nam*" and, on one occasion, signed "Namaste in advance"). A place where you might, at any given moment, be stuck with acupuncture needles simply because you mentioned you have a headache; where you are just as likely to be complimented on your aura as on your earrings. My colleagues and I hugged each other with alarming frequency, and people floated in for kundalini class all in white and with crystals stuck to their foreheads, and we *didn't* laugh at them. I have managed to maintain a professional tone when replying to an email about obtaining a guru (though my instinctive response – I am not ashamed to say – would have been 'How about you get a life?'), and kept a straight face through a 60 minute guidance session with a lovely lady who talks to the archangels, during which Gabriel himself advised me on my spiritual development and personal life. I won't lie to you: it wasn't always easy; there were times when I really struggled with all of this. I am a strange mixture of cynical and gullible, fluctuating between the two extremes but mostly settling somewhere along the way.

But, in a funny way, it's the extremes that keep me balanced. If I weren't reduced to hysterical laughter by a grown man banging on a tiny percussion instrument and instructing a class of forty to "receive the beautiful music", I would be too far gone. Equally, if I let my sarcasm loose whenever something rattled its cage, I would have missed out on a lot of wonderful, unexpected experiences, and would be pretty bad at my job, to boot. So I remain sceptical, but I'm open to everything. And I unequivocally believe that positive thinking works. And what's a moon ritual, when you strip it down to its essence, if not positive thinking? It goes by many different names, answers to assorted deities or forces and takes on a range of forms, but positive thinking is everywhere: from the most mystical of ancient philosophies all the way to 21st century pop culture; from the sacred texts of Hinduism to *The Secret* and its grandfather, *The Celestine Prophecy*; and from the yogic *sankalpa* to wiccan rituals to the prayers of Christianity to New Year Resolutions to birthday cake wishes. It all comes down to the same thing: setting an intention, focusing on what you want, and calling it to you. So yes, when someone tells me I can wave a crystal at the moon and ask for what I want, sure, I'll do it. Because I know it's not really about the ritual or the crystal or the moon; it's about me putting my soul into the things I want and opening the way for them to find me. And if that makes me a crazy new age fool, then so be it. I'm a crazy new age fool who's manifested a whole load of cool stuff. Including a free lunch, which I'm now going to sit down and enjoy, regardless of the ingredients.

It's been a month since the last full moon, and in that time I quit my job, left my flat in London, and moved to Athens for the summer. I remembered who I am, *all* of what I am, and I have been that person every day since. I am writing; I am staying up half the night to write. All these things are in line with what I asked for from the moon, and though the process was set in motion before the ritual, I don't believe the way it's all happening is coincidental. If you only believe in straight up cause and effect, you're not leaving any room for anything magical to happen. Like being true to yourself. Like writing. Like a man on your doorstep. And the man is no coincidence either; this man I manifested, who believes in manifestation, and who's also manifested me on his doorstep many times before. Who has stood beside me and will stand beside me again; who has waved me off on my journey, knowing that I'll come back when I'm ready. I asked for what I wanted, and this is what I got, and I've gotta trust the moon knows what it's doing, no matter how it chooses to go about it, because essentially it's just me, opening doors to a universe of infinite possibilities. Which is why I repeated the ritual the other night, with the full moon of May, on my mum's balcony in Athens. I stood there with my crystal, in my bare feet, and I greeted the moon like an old friend and the words came a lot easier this time because I know now that we have an understanding. And as I repeated the things I wanted, it occurred to me, as fact, that they were true. So I said it to the moon, *All these things are true*. And the moon nodded.

the unexpected papercuts of loss

This is a note about leaving. About all those tiny pockets of absence that it creates. Like the bubbles in an aero bar, leaving you hollow, somehow, a little insubstantial. I'm not talking about the huge gaping holes that it gouges into your life: your friends, the places you have loved, the routines and rituals that made up your everyday experience. Those are obvious, the expected consequences of any departure. Almost mundane. What I want to talk about is the collateral damage, all the little things that you're not quite entitled to mourn. A thousand unexpected papercuts of loss and longing, each one at most deserving of a wince, dismissible, but adding up, collectively, to quite a substantial amount of pain.

The background of the story is this: I spent the last two years working at a yoga centre in South West London, doing a job I absolutely loved. And then, two weeks ago, I left.

As a general rule, people who walk into a yoga centre are looking for something. And though we are not above the seasonal surges of post-holiday and pre-summer devotees, driven to yoga by New Year resolutions or the quest for that elusive bikini body, who generally sign up for whatever trial period is on offer, attend with varying degrees of enthusiasm and then drop off, and slink back into their previous routines with nothing more to show for it than yet another obsolete membership card in their wallets, yoga centres attract a steady trickle of newcomers all year round. Though we do, invariably, get some who stroll in and state, matter of factly, that they're looking to lose weight and tone their abs, and would we please direct them to the hardest, most dynamic classes (often causing the staff to shake their heads and smirk in a very un-yogic manner), most people who take those first, tentative steps into a yoga centre are brought here by something a lot less specific and a lot more profound than that. A loss, or a major event; a life changing incident or a tiny moment of realization, that the way they're living isn't quite working for them; an unnamed desire for something more, or a need for less. All equally valid. And it's in the nature of these places that those of us who work there have been attracted to yoga for the same reasons as the clients we are called upon to serve, and we cannot help but get involved. The boundaries between *us* and *them* are not so distinct as in other customer service roles. We are the gatekeepers of the yoga world, their guides in whichever quest has brought them here. We genuinely want them to find whatever they're looking for in yoga, and do our best to help them along their way.

Metta, loving kindness for ourselves and others, is at the core of a yogic way of life. We practice inversions and backbends to shift those stagnant fears that hold us back and open our hearts to give and receive love. And yet we are paradoxically warned against attachment. And therein lies the problem. How can I practice non-attachment without holding back? How can I put myself into another person, even for a few moments at a time, if I remain detached?

And so begin the papercuts. All those names I took the time to learn. The names I didn't use in conversation – despite what our customer service training manual prescribed (we're not above those, either) – but knew, nonetheless, and celebrated, along with the respective clients, when I could sign them into class without having to ask for their card. The details of their lives they shared, the things they chose to give me of themselves, little tokens of intimacy that I was fortunate enough to recognise as what they were, and kept them safe so I could bring them out next time, when they were needed. The daughter who told her ageing mum she wouldn't last a week. The husband who would really benefit from yoga but refused, point blank, to even try. The partner who was highly suspicious of his girlfriend's devotion to her weekly class, to the point that she had to pretend she was going out for drinks. The high-stress job, the sleepless nights, the upcoming wedding. Years of trying in vain to get pregnant; a miscarriage; the loneliness brought about by that 24 hour companion, the new baby. Chronic back pain. The fact that I could ask and, in the asking, make Ella or John or Katie feel that they belonged, that they mattered. And then: the daughter proven wrong. The husband talked into taking his first yoga class and begrudgingly admitting that he loved it. A full night's sleep; a whole day without pain. People turning up for class day after day, week after week, despite paranoid partners, cynical friends and unforgiving work schedules.

Papercuts. A toe stubbed on a chair leg. An elbow knocked into a doorway. Aicha, my fellow secret smoker, who talked to me like a friend and brought me chocolates for Christmas. Natalya, who came to me like a lost puppy brandishing a copy of the class schedule, and asked me to tell her exactly what to do; who followed my suggestions to the letter, and flourished, and made me feel like a guru superstar. Lucia, who told me about her friend that died of cancer, and sobbed in an empty yoga studio between classes, and let me put my arms around her. Elsa, who kept arriving after work, half-dead with exhaustion and determined to take two vinyasa classes in a row, and who actually trusted me when I said she needed rest more than yoga; who let me cover her with a blanket and watch over her as she slept, like a child, curled up on a bench bang in the middle of reception. And the pretty Indian girl, whose name I never knew, who confided in me about the constant chatter in her head – *'The blah-blah-blah, you know? All the time. Is it normal?'* – and gave me weekly reports as the voices were gradually reduced to whispers.

I am connected to these people and their stories, I am invested in their triumphs and their woes; I am attached. And yet they are only papercuts in the hierarchy of loss, and I am expected to just shrug them off and move on, because you don't cry over papercuts. Because, when you take a sober view to it, they are only clients that I served, and I'm just a girl with a name badge that signed them into class; it's debatable whether I'm even allowed to say goodbye.

Yoga teaches us the importance of letting go, of relinquishing the need to control, and trusting the universe to take us where we need to go. I made the decision to leave and I will stand by it and take the consequences as they come. I will fill the gaping holes with phone calls and emails and even old fashioned handwritten letters, and I will be OK because, ironically, the true friends we make along the way, the ones we ceremoniously say goodbye to when life takes us elsewhere, are the ones we'll never really be parted from. And my papercuts will heal, but I will remember every single person each one represents long after the sting has faded, long after I've forgotten all those names I painstakingly committed to memory. They all gave me the impossible gift of having been someone in their lives, a fellow traveller on their journeys, and I wouldn't have been in a position to receive it if I hadn't allowed myself to become attached.

Attachment is part of loving another person fully, and the pain that it potentially causes is a small price to pay for all that I have gained. I am an imperfect human being, flawed in a million different ways, but I have learned enough to know that I have a lot more to learn, and a very long way to go in this and every subsequent journey I undertake. And though I welcome it all, though I am willing to embrace everything that yoga has to teach, attachment is one thing I hope never to be cured from.

yoga for the pelvis

It started with a sore lower back and an unexpected lull in the treatments schedule on a nine-hour-shift Sunday in January. Siva, resident massage therapist and the universe's answer to every ache and pain a human body could care to invent, noticed me shifting my weight from foot to foot, in a vain attempt to release the tension.

'What's the matter, honey?' she said.

'Lower back,' I replied, pointing to the offending region.

Siva approached the desk behind which I stood, leaned in conspiratorially, and whispered: 'Can you sneak off for half an hour? I have no clients this afternoon.'

I could, as it happened. My break was coming up and, outside, London weather was doing what it does best, and raining misery upon its people; I had no umbrella, and no intention of exposing myself to such hostile conditions purely for the sake of fresh air.

'I'll be there as soon as I can,' I said.

(This, incidentally, is the job I *chose* to leave: where you were offered free massage treatments on your lunch break.)

A few minutes later, Siva had me lying face down on her double futon, in a candlelit treatment room between studios 2 and 3, where yoga classes were in progress, instructed me to relax, and did all kinds of magical and inexplicable things to my tension-riddled body. When the session came to an end, I wiped the dribble from my chin, straightened myself up as best as I could in preparation for returning to my post as the face (and hair) of a leading yoga centre, and enquired as to how damaged I actually was.

'You're very tight in your lower back,' Siva pronounced. 'And your hips.'

'Now you mention it,' I said, 'I've been feeling quite congested in that whole area.'

'Hmm.' Siva took a moment to consider. 'That's probably because you need some good sex.'

'I'm sorry?'

'Sex,' Siva repeated. 'For the pelvis, you know? It releases the tension. It might surprise you, but –'.

'It doesn't surprise me at all,' I confessed. 'I'm just surprised to hear you say it!'

Siva grinned. 'Well,' she said.

'I'll do what I can,' I promised. 'For the pelvis.'

'Exactly! That's what I say to my partner: do it for the pelvis!'

And thus, a catchphrase was born.

There are few things I enjoy more than a good euphemism. Also high on that list is turning the embarrassing moments of my life into anecdotes for the amusement of my friends. Siva had given me a great gift on both those counts. And I knew Laura would appreciate it more than most, so I rushed back to the reception desk, bursting with excitement, to share it with her.

'Hey,' she greeted me. 'How was your treatment?'

'Siva has just diagnosed me with needing sex!' And I recounted the tale. 'The pelvis,' I concluded, 'is not happy.'

'You'll need to address that,' Laura opined.

'Believe me,' I said, 'I'm trying!'

'Do it for the pelvis?' she suggested,

tentatively. Which was exactly the right thing to say.

'Do it for the pelvis!'

The pelvis, however, is very picky. Despite a couple of possibilities and applications from potential pelvis-pleasers, the pelvis and I both know that there is only one man it deems worthy of engaging with, and will not stoop so low as to even consider anyone else. Despite my assurances to Laura, I'm not really trying. At all. So it was a few months before I was able to make good on my promise to Siva, months during which Siva's gift was generously shared, and made it possible for my colleagues and I to casually and often very publicly discuss sex, or the lack thereof. Phrases like "the pelvis is frustrated" became common currency, so it was only natural that, when the happy incident occurred, I announced it by stating, apropos of nothing: 'The pelvis is delighted'. And all credit due to those present, who instantly rejoiced in the news (though the sex hair and dreamy look on my face may have been a bit of a giveaway).

This pelvis thing is like a goldmine: it just gives and gives and gives.

'My whole body aches,' I mentioned to Laura a couple of days later.

'What have you been doing?'

'Nothing!' I replied, earnestly. 'I haven't done any yoga for a couple of weeks. Except,' a pause, as the obvious answer occurred to me, 'yoga for the pelvis?'

Much amusement and giggling ensued, followed by fantasies of running a class entitled *Yoga for the Pelvis,* at which point it all got a bit weird and we composed ourselves and went back to work.

On another, separate occasion, my sister and I met one evening, when she had just returned from a dynamic vinyasa class and I from a particularly rigorous session of pelvic yoga. She was telling me how the teacher, Tony (who, incidentally, we both hero worship) had been in an especially relentless mood, and she demonstrated an advanced version of *Utthan Pristhasana,* Lizard Pose, that he had insisted upon. I tried to copy her, but she stopped me.

'You shouldn't do that,' she warned. 'You haven't done any hip openers.

'Actually...' I began, but then I thought better of it and said no more, not wanting to lower the tone with my distasteful jokes, though I was privately quite amused. If my sister noticed the self-satisfied smirk that escaped me, she was kind enough not to bring it up.

All those evolutions of the pelvis euphemism, however, got me thinking about the connection between yoga and sex. Though it is possible to perform them mechanically, a mindful approach is beneficial in both practices. The experience of sex, like yoga, is significantly enhanced if you immerse yourself fully in the present moment. The *mula bandha* certainly comes into it; and if it doesn't, it really, *really* should! Then come the aforementioned hip openers, as well as backbends, inversions and twists, and maybe even a few stray dogs, some of which actually do face down. Affirmations, often expressed loudly and enthusiastically, feature in both, as does breathwork — though the yogic version is arguably a lot more controlled. There is also the spiritual dimension, the element of communion with the divine, which was brought to my attention recently. During one session which the pelvis evidently found very much to its liking, I heard myself repeatedly taking the Lord's name in vain – *oh god, oh god, oh my god!* – and paused for a moment to ponder this. 'I don't even believe in God,' I remarked. The man in question, The One The Pelvis Chose, smiled, taking this as a compliment. Which it was. Especially coming from an absolute pedant such as myself, who won't even capitalise the word "god", in case it is mistaken for piety. And, finally, no one can deny the similarities between a closing *savasana* and the post-coital nap. Except that the former generally involves significantly more clothing.

None of this, of course, is new, and I'm sure the tantric tradition can provide a much more coherent and philosophically rooted explanation of the inherent bonds between yoga and sex. These are just the scattered thoughts of a reluctant yogi, inspired by a semi-regular yoga practice, a pelvic euphemism, and some good sex – just as Siva prescribed. But, in practicing yoga for the pelvis, I have rediscovered sex as a noble and spiritual pursuit, which, I am pleased to report, is completely in line with one of the most valuable lessons I've learned so far: yoga doesn't need to be confined to the studio; it can be a part of everything you do. You can practice yoga while walking down the street, or waiting for the bus, or doing your shopping. And, I can now confidently add, you can practice yoga during sex. All it takes is a bit of awareness, a tiny mental shift, and – bam! –*everything is yoga.*

As long as it keeps the pelvis happy; that's the important thing.

***

The pelvis is currently taking a short break from yoga, and bearing this in a brave and stoical manner. Thanks for asking.

what moron?

This is an actual conversation:
>'Rude yogis is an oxymoron.'
>'*What* moron?'

Oxymoron is an excellent word. Defined as a combination of contradictory or incongruous words, it derives from the ancient Greek *oxys* (sharp, keen) and *moros* (dull, stupid), making the word oxymoron an oxymoron in itself.
>Cruel to be kind.
>Deafening silence.
>Old news
>Clearly misunderstood.
>Rude yogis.

The problem with rude yogis is the illusions most of us harbour about the yoga world and those that populate it. We expect practitioners, and even more so teachers, to be slightly more evolved than the general public. We expect certain fundamental values of the yogic philosophy to frame all of our interactions. Humility. Non competitiveness. Awareness. A little bit less of the ego, a little bit more of the loving kindness.

But the yoga world is, in fact, the world, with yoga mats thrown in. And, yes, it does contain some incredible, inspiring, enlightened people, but not exclusively. It also contains people who are only just embarking upon this journey, people who have taken a wrong turn somewhere along the way, people who have completely misread not only the map but the entire situation, and have arrived at some very un-yogic places, fully kitted out in their lululemon leggings and sipping the obligatory green smoothie. It contains people who are stressed, lonely, depressed, in pain; people who are doing their best but, actually, they've had a terrible day at work. People who are, quite frankly, arseholes, and no amount of yoga will change that.

Before I stumbled into a job in the yoga world, I worked in pubs for years, and there is no oxymoron in rude drunks. The pub world is very clean cut: the separation between *us* and *them* is absolute, two different tribes at war, and the bar is a battlefield, every night. You *expect* difficult customers, and they never disappoint. Rudeness is standard, and physical violence is a very real possibility. In my time as a barmaid, casually ducking out of the way as bottles were tossed in my general direction became almost routine, and people have threatened to glass me on more occasions than I care to recall. (I love the fact that the English language actually contains the verb *to glass*: "to hit someone (usually in the face or head) with a pint glass", by the way.)

But then you cross into a world that's softly lit by candles and scented by incense and benevolent deities smile down upon you, and it puts you under a spell, and you forget. It's customer service, sure, but it's *yoga*. When asked, during my interview, why I thought I was suitable to work at a yoga centre (an interview which, incidentally, took place in a pristine white studio, where the manager, supervisor and I sat barefoot on purple bolsters on the floor), the argument I supplied was: 'This is my happy place.' Complete with manic smile.

Susanne, the manager, regarded me curiously, obviously trying to decide whether I was dangerous or merely deluded. 'You know it's a job, right?' she said. 'You know it's not easy.'

'Sure,' I replied. 'But it's *yoga*.'

Susanne and Caroline, the supervisor, exchanged a knowing look. I would learn.

And learn I did, but it was hard. The first time it happens is deeply shocking, and though the intensity does lessen with exposure, you never quite get used to it. Every encounter with a rude yogi takes you by surprise. This is the danger with always wanting to see the best in people: sometimes they have no best to show you. But you have to remain open to it; you learn to protect yourself, to an extent, but then you let your guard down again, every time.

Enter the high-maintenance Ashtangi – let's call her Judy – who left her shampoo and body lotion in the changing rooms, came back a week later to discover they'd been thrown away in our weekly lost property clear-out, and accused us of having stolen them. When I assured her that none of my colleagues were thieves, she snorted in disbelief; when I explained what had actually happened, she informed me I was a liar. She used other choice words, too, in a lengthy rant delivered at the reception desk, and then got into a habit, on subsequent visits, of telling everyone in the changing rooms that the staff were thieves, and leaving notes, headed "Dear fellow yogi", warning against leaving property unattended. Lisa, who worked herself up into a frenzy over a booking error, attacked my colleague and I personally while we desperately tried to figure it out, and nearly decked me when I made the mistake of touching her on the shoulder. Kirsten, who famously flashed another colleague the finger when reminded not to use her phone, and then defended this gesture when I, trembling all over, confronted her about it. And Derek, whose rage over being asked, for health and safety reasons, to please refrain from practising in the studio unsupervised, escalated – via a barrage of random, spittle-enhanced insults – into racist comments directed specifically at me, all justified in the name of the "spiritualism" that was, apparently, lacking in my attitude. And, of course, the endless, nameless clients who gave us abuse, daily, on account of being refused entry into classes that had already started, or were full.

Kirsten apologised for her behaviour that same evening. Lisa did not, but she was a completely transformed person on her next visit, and every time she's come in since. The way she approaches the desk, so timidly, smiling the sweetest, most humble smile, makes me want to hug her, but I'm still a little scared of touching her, so I don't. Derek is an irredeemable bully, and he was banned from the centre; he did not take it in the spirit of spiritualism at all. And Judy – a different kind of bully – was offered free classes, in a gesture of good will that she did not return: she still warns fellow yogis darkly about the dangers of unattended property, and pointedly blanks me, the liar, on her every visit. Judy has no fellows in this world, yogic or otherwise.

Perhaps there is no oxymoron here, after all. Perhaps there are no rude yogis, just people who happen to do yoga and are rude. Perhaps what makes a yogi is not so much the things they do in class, but the way they choose to behave out of it, in the real world. So you may never do a headstand, but if yoga teaches you to be a little kinder, a little more patient, to see the good in people despite what they actually show you, then you're more of a yogi than Judy will ever be. And as for me, I've been called a lot of things, but I'd rather be a moron than an oxymoron, no matter how much I love the word.

#hypocrite

A couple of months ago, I didn't even know what a hashtag *was*. I consider myself quite a tech-savvy person, perhaps not exactly at the vanguard of the latest developments, but certainly not lagging behind, either. But hashtags defeated me. Overnight, the entire world was inundated by the bloody things. To me, the # symbol still stood for "number", as in #1. It also served as punctuation in automated phone menus, as in: "type in your account number and then press the hash key". Now it inexplicably appeared on all of my friends' posts, followed by seemingly random words. I was completely baffled; I had to look it up. Once fully up to date, I snorted in derision whenever someone posted a photo of their child followed by #baby, and declared, with utter confidence, that I would never use a hashtag.

Flash forward to May 2014, and all of a sudden I'm the Queen of the social media, and I can hashtag with the best of them. I have three facebook pages, two twitter accounts, one blog, two websites, two accounts on instagram and I am also on Google+. I am a slave to likes, hits, views, retweets and the refresh button on my browser. I need more followers. Facebook informs me, ominously, that my post reach is down by 25,4% from the previous week, while Google Analytics reports that my site was accessed by one person in India, using Chrome on a Mac. Is it all getting a little out of hand?

I recently took my life apart – the life in London that I

knew and loved – to make space for writing. I quit my job, put my stuff in storage, packed my laptop and a few pairs of shorts and relocated to my mum's flat in Athens, to spend the next four months being a writer. So far, so noble. And though artistic and spiritual pursuits are an end in themselves, and being true to yourself is a non-negotiable condition for being a happy and giving member of society, we'd all like to earn a living doing what we love. Finding perfect alignment in your *Virabhadrasana II* or producing beautiful, thought-provoking prose may be wonderfully fulfilling, but it doesn't pay the rent. The fact is, if you want to make it as a freelance anything, you have to play the PR game. And PR is, ultimately, all about egos. Egos *in competition*, all clamouring for attention. *Please like me*; like me *more* than other people. And *followers*? Seriously? Whatever happened to readers, to students? Even the vocabulary we have adopted is wrong. It makes my stomach turn, just thinking about it.

But I'm a hypocrite, and owning up to it doesn't make it less so. When I set up a facebook page for *This Reluctant Yogi*, I introduced it by saying: "Needy alter ego. Please like." I thought I was making a stand by pointing out that I was aware of the irony inherent in promoting a page dedicated to yoga. But where I actually stood was slap bang in the middle of a game I had self-righteously excused myself from. If you were to type in #hypocrite, my name wouldn't come up, but it should.

Writers get a bit of leeway: we are not bound by any particular moral code; our only responsibility is to produce good writing and as long as we do that we can get away with being a bit obnoxious. But yoga practitioners

41

and, even more so, yoga teachers are expected to embody the values they advocate. And yet the yoga world is rife with guru complexes and superstar teachers and, as the recent yoga selfie debate has highlighted, encourages competition even as it tells us that yoga is non-competitive. But of course these people have bills to pay, just like the rest of us, and trusting in Ganesh alone won't cut it. They need full classes and workshops booked up months in advance and DVDs and books and branded merchandise. They need to strike a balance somewhere between noble destitution and #hypocrite, between selling and selling out.

For me, in my dual capacity as writer and yogi, it all came to a head a couple of weeks ago, when I had an article published on Elephant Journal. The initial excitement quickly gave way to anxiety, as I found myself welded to my computer for two days straight, compulsively pressing refresh to check whether my views had reached the 2,000 mark (whereupon, I was told, the article would be moved to the front page of the journal). My views stagnated at around 1,000, and I was disappointed. And it occurred to me, as I lamented my lack of likes (needy alter ego indeed) and kept a jealous eye on other articles whose views soared to tens of thousands, that this was insane. *One thousand people.* When a week ago I would have been happy with fifty. One thousand people read my words, and the fact that I didn't immediately recognise that as the small miracle that it was meant that something had gone horribly wrong. And I had just wasted two days that I could have spent writing, or thinking, or doing yoga. I had failed in my responsibilities as both writer and yogi, all in the name of being *liked.*

Being aware of the irony isn't enough, nor does it absolve us of the responsibilities we've willingly undertaken. But maybe it's a start. Anyone who knows me knows of my ongoing battle with the concept of non-attachment as it applies to human relationships, but perhaps it's appropriate in this context. Perhaps the way to handle our roles as PR managers and social media bitches is to be a little less attached to the outcome of our campaigns. To take it all a little less seriously, to laugh at ourselves as we do it. To play the game, but remember that it's a game we're playing. And when we're finished playing, to go back to the things that brought us here in the first place: to writing, to thinking, to doing yoga. To being who we are. To being liked by very few people, loved by fewer still, but genuinely: for our true, hashtag-free selves, followed by no one, but following our hearts.

***

You are, of course, encouraged to follow me on facebook, twitter and instagram (ironically).

do you know who i am?

Every Monday, at 8 am, Takako comes to clean the yoga mats in Studio 1. She takes them out of the cupboard, one by one, and spreads them out in neat rows across the studio floor, and then she sprays each one with a mixture of water and tea tree oil and wipes them down with a towel, top to bottom, with sweeping, circular motions. While she waits for them to dry, she moves on to the jumble of scrunched up purple blankets, piled up high and precariously and threatening an avalanche at any given moment; she shakes these out and then folds them into precise rectangles before stacking them up on the shelf, in perfect purple towers of order. Takako performs all these rituals slowly, and in complete silence. Once the mats have dried, she kneels down in front of each one, folding her body deeply over it, eyes closed, as if in prayer, and everything is stillness except her hands working expertly, rhythmically, to roll every mat into a tight, immaculate coil. At this point, people start arriving for the 9 am hot yoga class, swooshing the door open, anxious to lay their mats down and get on with their day. They don't understand what they've walked into; they have no concept of the sanctity of what they're witnessing. I always wish they'd take a moment to look, but they don't. All they see is a tiny, silent girl, rolling mats up on her hands and knees. Takako never rushes, and never looks up. She completes her task, gathers her things and drifts out of the studio, like dust blown away by the breeze – unnoticed, unheard. She is a volunteer; she does all this week after week, in exchange for yoga. I have never seen her take a class, but if you asked me to define what a yog is, I would invite you to watch Takako clean the mats on a Monday morning. And that may be the best answer I could give you.

For a while, I had the best job in the world. Five days a week, I strolled along the Thames and over Battersea Bridge to arrive at a yoga centre in Chelsea, where, in my uniform of bare feet and purple top, I wondered around serenely, making the place look pretty. I tidied up the props in the studios. I rearranged the flyers on the front desk in neat stacks. I made sure the candles were lit and the incense never stopped burning. I artfully arranged fresh flowers in the multiple hands of softly-lit deities. I cleaned the mats so that my fellow yogis could enjoy a hygienic and sweetly-scented practice, rather than *ujai*-inhaling the odour of other people's feet (my secret being the addition of a few drops of orange essential oil to the antibacterial and antiviral blend of tea tree and lemon). I removed tangles of hair from the shower drains. I kept the sinks clean and the toilet paper stocked up. I dusted. I took the rubbish out. I smiled.

I performed all these menial tasks with a sense of apprenticeship, an echo of Master Miyagi's wipe on/wipe off method of training in *The Karate Kid*. I didn't take the job to learn lessons about humility, but it came naturally, and my cynical, reactive self conceded some truths about impermanence, which I would have rejected outright had they been delivered in any other way, as my beautifully rolled up mats were unfurled and stepped on with dirty feet and my gleaming sinks were splashed with scummy water. I revelled in the meditative quality of the most repetitive chores, and surrendered to the endless cycle of

45

chaos-order-chaos that my job entailed. I came to appreciate the subtle math of all these little things I did adding up to a place that people loved.

My official job title was "Centre Assistant" but on our company-wide contact sheet I was inexplicably listed as "Chelsea Centre Cleaner". This title survived numerous updated versions of the document, as people came and went and changed positions within the company, and even persisted when I started taking on Front of House shifts, and was eventually promoted to supervisor. We laughed about this, my colleagues and I. 'Where's Chelsea Centre Cleaner?' they would say, and I would appear and declare myself at their service. Occasionally, people took it upon themselves to correct this slight on my honour, crossing out the offending job title and graffitiing compliments next to my name. But I wasn't offended. I loved what I did, and it made no difference what anybody called me.

People did sometimes make assumptions about me – my abilities, my prospects, my level of education – based on the tasks they saw me perform. Sweeping the studio floor, wiping the sinks, dusting the shelves where they left their shoes. Their regard for me decreased when I was called upon to unblock a toilet, and increased, marginally, when I proved myself able to advise them on which type of yoga to practice. It completely baffled them when they demanded to see the supervisor and I would stand up, duster in hand, and go 'That'll be me', unable to fathom that I could be many things at once. I won't lie to you: there were moments when someone would push me too far, and my ego would pipe and roar *"Do you know who I am?*" and I wanted to shove my degrees in their smug, ignorant faces; those were the moments when Chelsea Centre Cleaner stung a bit. But they were moments and they would pass and – after a brief interlude of swearing in the office – I would soon remember that other people's perceptions of me were merely reflections of who they were, and I would only be cast in the light of their preconceptions if I placed myself there. So I'd get back on my hands and knees, and happily carry on picking up bits of rubbish off the floor while they trotted around, above me, in designer shoes that Chelsea Centre Cleaner could never afford. And there were other moments, too, when somebody would notice me wiping the sink after I'd washed my hands, and do the same. When somebody would take the time to help me put the props away after class. When somebody would come up to me and say 'It makes a difference what you do. Thank you.' The little things. Adding up.

The first summer I was there, I had to go away for almost a month, and we found someone to replace me in my absence. She came to do a shift with me, to learn the job. As I enthusiastically demonstrated how to polish the chrome fittings in the bathrooms, she took a step back and fixed me with a look of utter disdain.

'So this is a cleaning job,' she said, flatly.

'There's quite a lot of cleaning, yes.' I smiled.

'So basically you're telling me that I'm a *cleaner*,' she insisted.

I shrugged. 'I don't know *what* you are,' I replied, truthfully. 'That's up to you. All I'm telling you is that this is my job and I love it.' I tilted my head to admire my handiwork. 'Look!' I said, to enforce my point. 'Look at my shiny sink!'

She shook her head, her face a mixture of horror and pity. 'I hope,' she said slowly, 'in the next four weeks I don't end up like you.'

She didn't. She ended up with a job she hated, and she did it badly, with an air of contempt designed to show that she was made for better things, but which only served to keep her apart, and unliked. Upon leaving, she went to India, to complete her teacher training and spend six months in an Ashram. Where cleaning other people's shit is *spiritual*, whereas in Chelsea it's just plain demeaning. This person is now a yoga teacher. She's more than happy to lecture you about *dharma* and the yoga *sutras* and wave the *Hatha Yoga Pradipika* in your face, but she won't stoop so low as to polish a tap. Go figure.

I think that everyone should clean a few toilets. And if you're into meditation, try rolling up a hundred belts in an empty studio on a Wednesday afternoon. If you want to learn about letting go, try standing there, immediately after, and watching as forty people bustle in and unroll them again, so casually. Before you start using big words, try mastering the little things, the ones that go unnoticed. You may find that they add up to more than you expected. And take a moment to think about a Japanese girl cleaning mats for the love of it.

Our contact sheet was updated a couple of months before I left. Someone, somewhere, finally noticed and changed my job title to "Supervisor". I felt a little sad, but then I thought perhaps the universe had decided my apprenticeship was complete. But that's a dangerous statement to make and, as I move on to other things, I'll keep the original version of that sheet pinned up on a board in my mind, to help me remember what the world looks like from that perspective, what it feels like to look up at people without feeling like they're looking down on you. Because the answer is *no*. They don't know who I am. But I do: I am Chelsea Centre Cleaner. Please address me by my proper title.

the conditions for unconditional love

I've been thinking about love a lot lately. My sister is getting married this weekend, and I am going to be her witness, and sign my name on a document officially declaring her and Arek husband and wife (or the other way round, as the case may be). And this makes me feel happy and grateful and proud and a little in awe. But, my own role in this event aside, my bearing witness, both officially and unofficially, to what is truly and unequivocally an excellent thing, I cannot help but question the purpose of such declarations. Weddings, marriages, and their necessity in connection to love.

My sister and I are not wedding people. In fact, the mere mention of the topic as it relates to our own lives is likely to cause, in both of us, an almost phobic reaction. In addition to this, we share a – partly justifiable – mistrust of marriage itself, as exemplified by our parents and society at large. The phonecall in which she announced to me the fact of her engagement could be described, without exaggeration, as one of the happiest and most awkward conversations two people have ever had. We have never talked about weddings; we have never fantasised, as other girls, of dresses and engagement rings. This was a foreign land, full of dragons and booby traps, and we circumnavigated these terrors as best we could, to arrive, clumsily, at a mutual conclusion of joy. We weren't trying to be obscure, or unconventional; we just don't have the vocabulary for this sort of thing. None of us really do.

And yet we try. We try, with words, to explain why people get married, to define a marriage, to express love. To capture its essence, to measure it, quantify it, evaluate it – demystify it, perhaps, to make it more manageable, more attainable. We are, as a society, entirely preoccupied with love, endlessly producing quotes, metaphors, clichés and contradictions. They're in our art and our literature, our everyday conversations, our highbrow theories and our pop songs. And, regardless of whether we subscribe to fairytale endings or take the cynical view and reject love and marriage outright, in our moments of elation and of pain we all drunkenly sing along.

And if you turn to Eastern philosophies in search of a more sober perspective, as I have, it gets even more confusing. The teachings of Buddhism encourage loving kindness and compassion, yet discourage attachment, while Buddhist monks are happy to bless a union that is basically a marriage by another name. The Buddha is quoted as having said: "He who loves fifty people has fifty woes; he who loves no one has no woes." And I don't understand whether this is a warning or simply a statement of fact; whether those woes are to be avoided, or accepted – welcomed, even – as a part of love.

It is then suggested that we *should* love, but love all creatures *equally*. And I don't think that's possible, sustainable or even desirable. I can see the virtue in approaching each person and each situation with love; it takes practice, but it can be done, and I call that *kindness*. But to enact love, *to love*, as a verb, is a different thing entirely and I, for one, cannot produce that level of emotion for everyone I meet.

And further: love, in its truest, purest form, should be *unconditional*. And sometimes it is. But the reason it became love, the reason it grew into love is because certain conditions were in place when it began. Conditions as in *circumstances* rather than *terms*, but conditions, nonetheless. Does this negate its unconditional nature, retroactively, once it reaches that stage? Perhaps I'm taking things too literally, and this is just another case of our vocabulary letting us down, but it seems to me that for all their dogma, these philosophies are placing conditions on who and how I love.

But *love is not possession*: this one I can live with. Yet I have lain in a man's arms and felt, with my whole, entire self: "I am yours. You are mine." And it has nothing to do with ownership, but with the fact that something in the way this universe moves has brought us together and that's exactly where we should be. A place where all the definitions of love cease to matter. But when I try to explain it, these are the words that come out. They're the only words I have.

But what does all of this say about marriage? Does a wedding validate a love? Is placing a ring on someone's finger a declaration of ownership? Is it, as Beyonce suggests in the eloquent lyric "If you liked it then you shoulda put a ring on it", all about staking a claim? I think in many cases, in many marriages, it is. I may find the notion of ownership incompatible with my understanding of love, but to many people, the idea of belonging to someone, of someone belonging to them, is an arrival, a homecoming – it's where they want to be. Just like I want to be in that place of stillness and certainty that I have found lying next to a man I love, and most marriages are lands I never want to visit.

But there are other marriages. Ones where love needs no validation. Where commitment transcends the signing of papers, if papers have been signed at all. It depends on where you place yourself in this equation. You can stand next to someone, or you can follow them, or you can lead the way. You can stand next to someone and place a ring on your own finger, not a promise to anyone else, but a symbol for yourself, for how *you* feel. You can get married, or you can marry; you can be a passive or an active part of the grammar that makes up your relationship. You can have a marriage where nobody belongs to anybody else but perhaps, if you're lucky, you belong together. And you can hold their hand, but loosely; if they want to go away, they will, no matter how tightly you grip.

Words, grammar, syntax. Xs and Ys and the mathematical formulas that bring them together. The laws of physics, the laws of nature. Symbols and signatures, rings and vows and altars. Faith, fate, god and endless theories. We summon all these things to try and explain the inexplicable, to express something that defies expression, as elusive as it is ever-present, as abstract as it is tangible, as extraordinary as it is commonplace; something that slips through your fingers like your lover's hand when you squeeze too tight, but will happily settle in your open palm if you know enough to hold it out, and wait. And it's the human condition that we keep trying, that we will always keep trying, because if there ever comes a day when we stop trying, it will mean we have captured something that shouldn't be caught, demystified the mystery that keeps our lives in motion. And that, I think, will be the day that everything stops. That will be the day when saying the words "I love you" will express exactly what we mean, and I cannot think of anything sadder than that.

There is no such thing as a universal marriage, just as there's no universal definition of love. Those are choices we make, each of us, for ourselves, and saying you don't believe in marriage is not an ideology, it's a cop out. Love no one. Have no woes.

I still think my sister is very brave, and there'll be dragons to slay (or approach with love, and convert to household pets), but I'm not worried. I have every reason to believe that she and Arek will have one of those other marriages, the ones that don't make me want to run away screaming. I think they have it already. Because neither of them is getting married: both are marrying the person they love. Because, at times when I've lost my faith, I've looked to them and seen that they have built their life in that same place of stillness and certainty, and though they may wander off sometimes, they always know how to get back. Because they've shown me that big love doesn't necessarily equal big drama, and when you're faced with it, you might no longer need to put it into words.

But words are sometimes all we have, and mine are all I have to give. So this is dedicated to them: in hope, in admiration, and in love. Not equal, but as unconditional as it comes.

sometimes the answer is not coconut oil

For close to twenty years now, my friend Eileen and I have shared a common fear, and its name is *whale music*. Ever since our teens, whenever one of us strays too far into the realm of the new agey, the other will warn darkly: "You're gonna turn into one of those people who listen to whale music." And that will normally suffice to pull the offending party back from the brink of the abyss.

Devised in the mid- to late-nineties, when we first became aware of our proclivity for bullshit and its dangerous connotations, the term *whale music*, a.k.a. recordings of whale song and other nature sounds, stands for everything that is wrong with the world. Examples of whale music behaviours include, but are not limited to: giving vague and soul-searching answers to simple questions such as "how are you?"; smelling permanently of incense; commenting on people's auras, unconsulted; discussing your chakras; attributing personal challenges, weather phenomena and the traffic on the King's Road to "cosmic events"; sitting on the floor, in the lotus position, when there are perfectly good chairs around and everybody else is using them; claiming to be "spiritual"; using the word *Namaste* at any time outside of yoga class; and, of course, actually listening to recordings of whale song and other nature sounds, for pleasure.

The fear of whale music kept us relatively safe throughout our teens and most of our twenties. Which is a small miracle, given that we both started our adult lives as art students in late nineties London, shared a flat whose furnishings were almost exclusively comprised of items scavenged from the streets and draped artfully with multicoloured, tie-dye throws, hung out with people whose conversation revolved entirely around the meaning of life, and were attracted to men with unwashed hair and painted toenails. And that we burned a lot of incense.

But we got through it, somehow. Eileen grew up, got married, had kids and discovered she had no time for lighting incense, much less for reclining on cushions embroidered with the OM symbol and pondering her spiritual development. I, in the meantime, fell in love with a man who is likely to use the phrase "living in the present moment" in any given conversation, even when the conversation is about what we're having for dinner. (It's a skill.) And then fell sideways into the world of yoga, and got a job which involved lighting incense and tending to statues of Hindu deities for a living.

Have I become one of those people, Eileen? Would you tell me if I had? If you were to take an inventory of my room, you would find: three Buddha statues (one of which is plastic, battery-operated, and glows red and pink and purple and green), two of Ganesh, two hand-painted incense holders, one aromatherapy oil diffuser, a large number of candles and tea lights, and one inspirational quote card reminding me that "I am perfectly adequate for all situations". My yoga mat, purple, is rolled up in a corner by my bed. I own a quartz crystal and use it, monthly, to harness the energy of the full moon. I have a daily yoga practice and have even referred to it as that, albeit self-consciously, on several occasions. On my computer, I have music playlists entitled "OM", "Love Life / Live Yoga" and, to my shame, "Sounds of Serenity". My kitchen cupboard is an absolute treasure trove of the latest superfoods. I make my own keffir, daily. When faced with adversity, I am likely to take a deep breath, smile, and say something infuriatingly positive such as "The Universe will provide". And my answer to everything is either "yoga" or "coconut oil". Or both. Have I become a kinder, happier person, better equipped to handle my own life and be of service to others? Or is it all just so much whale music?

I'm all for spiritual development. I'm all for awareness and mindfulness and loving kindness. Looking after yourself, mind, body and spirit. It would be lovely if we all spoke a little softer, if we took a little longer to think before we act. If we were all a little enlightened. The world would be a better place. Like the tote bag I carry on my shoulder proclaims: *Yoga will save the world*.

But who will save us from whale music? Who will be there to remind us, gently, that we're taking it a bit too far? When our facebook feeds are inundated by inspirational quotes and we've lost the ability to say things in our own words. When gluten is the devil and eating cake is tantamount to suicide. When we boast, daily, of our dietary restrictions and post snapshots of ourselves in the course of a practice that was designed to be personal. When every yoga class is an opportunity to open our hearts, to acknowledge the pain, the frustration, the sadness within, to welcome it, to *go with it*. When we consult spiritual healers and gurus and medicine men and forget to talk to our friends. When we ostensibly strive for balance, and fail to notice the irony of seeking it in extremes.

I cannot be the only one who's getting a bit tired of this.

It's wonderful that you've discovered your true purpose in life, and that your soul is blooming, much like a lotus flower, in the light of your new-found awareness, but sometimes, when I ask how you are, I'm just looking for "fine". Sometimes the universe does not provide. Sometimes I feel like shit and that's the thing I want to acknowledge. Sometimes I don't want to do yoga, although I have the time and I know it'll make me feel better. I drink four cups of coffee a day. As I draw my yoga practice to a close, I bow my head, say *Namaste*, and smoke a cigarette. When I give massages, I light candles and burn essential oils and use my special therapist voice to urge my clients to relax, but often skip the "Sounds of Serenity" playlist in favour of the Beastie Boys. I'm more than happy to discuss yoga philosophy over dinner, but I'll be eating steak and chips. And I might have cake for dessert. And then I'll go home and cover myself head to toe in coconut oil, give a nod to Ganesh, and settle in bed to read my book about mindfulness. And somewhere therein, between cigarette smoke and Nag Champa incense, between the Beastie Boys and whale music, I find my balance.

Sometimes the answer is not coconut oil. Eileen and I went to the beach the other day. As she sensibly applied sun block to her face and shoulders, I quoted an article I'd read the day before, and informed her that we had, as a society, become obsessed with sun protection, to the detriment of our vitamin D production, when, in actual fact, we needed exposure to the sun more than we needed protecting from it. And that I, for one, had only applied a thin layer of coconut oil to my face, which has a natural

SPF of 4. At home that evening, I noticed an unfamiliar tingling sensation in my cheeks, along with an uncomfortable tightness. I put my hands to my face; it felt a little tender to the touch. I was completely baffled: I, of extra-dark Mediterranean complexion, had never experienced this sort of thing before. I stood in front of the mirror, did a double take at the red, glowing thing that had become of my face (not unlike my battery-operated Buddha), and laughed. I smothered myself in coconut oil (it does work on sunburn), and called Eileen.

'I got sunburn!' I confessed.

'Hmm,' she said politely. 'Despite the coconut oil?'

And just like that, she pulled me back from the brink, once again. Without having to say the words. Back to a place where I was just a shamefaced, red-faced idiot and my friends liked me, regardless. In the distance, a whale sung sadly as it swam away, towards people more spiritually evolved than us.

Don't heed the siren song of whales. Go to yoga class. Look after your soul. Open your heart and go with whatever you find in there – but try not to go too far. Eat raw leaves if you must, but remember to find your balance somewhere. Eileen and I will be sitting in the shade, wearing our SPF 30, and sipping our iced coffee as we ponder how much sand her children can eat before we need to stop them. I'll be discreetly working on my *Mula Bandha* while I smoke a cigarette. Join us. We can talk about our *chakras,* if you like.

beat on the brat

There seems to be a trend for yogi-bashing lately. I completely understand. There has been many a time when I've felt the urge to bash a yogi myself. But that's a very big, heavy stick you're wielding, and I'm not sure you know how to use it. Or why.

One of the most recent examples of yogi-bashing is Naomi McAuliffe's article in the *Guardian*. Entitled *I'm with Father O'Baoill,* the opening paragraph reports on how a Catholic priest warned his parishioners that yoga is an unsavoury activity that may endanger their souls, and goes on to mention other cases when the Church has expressed ignorant or downright bigoted opinions about yoga, on the basis of its "spirituality". I'll add another example: a few years back, an Orthodox priest, the Bishop of a large metropolitan area in Athens, Greece, launched a direct attack against yoga in general and yoga centres in his jurisdiction in particular, and issued an official statement to that effect, employing phrases such as "demonic dogma", "denial of the Faith" and "blasphemy against the Holy Spirit" to terrify his flock and protect their immortal souls. And a lot of people agreed with him.

So, *the Church is a bit narrow-minded*. Sad? Yes. It's sad that an organisation that yields such power should still be using its influence so irresponsibly, and demonstrating such insecurity in its own values and such lack of faith in its members. If your status as a good Christian is threatened by engaging in a few downward dogs and relieving your chronic back ache, then it's a very fragile construction and no amount of terror-monging will keep it from crashing down. It's sad. But shocking? No. This is nothing new. What's new, however, is that there are now priests who do yoga, because they know their souls are theirs to give to whomever they want. And that's tremendously reassuring, both because yoga is finally moving out of the realm of the mystical and the elite and becoming more accessible, and because we are gradually, as a society, stretching our minds to include possibilities that didn't seem available in the not so distant past.

But let's move on to yogi-bashing, as Naomi promptly does for the remainder of her article. Using Father O'Baoill's description of yoga as an "unsavoury activity" as a launching pad for a number of badly-sketched stereotypes, Naomi goes on to explain, in a manner that readers are supposed to recognise as "tongue-in-cheek" and humorous, the reasons why she is in agreement. What seems to bother Naomi most about yogis – a.k.a. people "who need supernatural stories in order to get bendy" – is their smugness, which goes hand-in-hand with their insistence on telling you all about their practice, the "floppy" clothes they wear, and their feet. There is also a bizarre and – in my view – dangerous allusion to how "these people rarely drink alcohol", which, apparently, only highlights how boring they are. But the fascinating thing is not the article itself, but the responses it's elicited. There are, at the latest count, 879 comments, with more still being added, almost a week after its publication. Some are actually very funny, but the vast majority are either extremely vitriolic and narrow-minded or extremely defensive and ineffective. I spent close to an hour reading them; I couldn't stop. And then I promised myself I wouldn't respond. But I just cannot resist.

Having had a couple of days to think about it, however, I will attempt to respond to the Naomis and the yoga bashers of this world without falling into the trap that makes even the most well-meaning yoga defenders sound, well, *defensive*, and deserving of the widely-held view that yogis have no sense of humour. And the trap is taking it personally. There is absolutely no use in pointing out how you, in fact, go for a pint after every yoga class, for which you wear H&M leggings, and have a very good sense of humour, thanks very much. Stereotypes are not about individuals, and generalisations are just a giant net cast by people who are vaguely pissed off at something but lack either the skill or the insight to identify exactly what it is. Or the courage to admit it.

So what is it, exactly, about yogis that pisses you off so much? The smugness? Sure, many yogis are insufferably smug. Some are irritating to the point of GBH. But so are many new mothers, office workers, indoor rowing fanatics and people who make omelettes, and they, too, talk ceaselessly about their respective pursuits and post related photos on facebook. And unless you're prepared to tell me that you're fascinated by every single photo of her dribbling infant that some girl you went to college with twenty years ago insists on sharing with the world, or that the status updates by your former colleague who lives in Scarborough about her nightly drinks with the girls in their local are an important public service, then I really don't see why it's the yogis who are getting all the shit. But, funnily enough, you don't often come across articles attacking new mothers for being excited about their babies, or criticising them for wearing nursing bras. Cause that wouldn't be cool.

But it's a fact that I cannot deny: yogis like to talk about yoga. A lot. When I get together with my yogi friends, that's precisely what we do. Just like we talk about sex and books and food and our jobs, and anything else that occupies large parts of our everyday lives. But I'll make you a deal: as soon as you give me a good reason for not discussing mutual interests with my friends, I will stop immediately. As long as you also stop talking about fashion, or art, or politics, or your children, or whatever it is that you and your friends find interesting. How does that sound?

In the meantime, however, let's look at this rationally: if you're being exposed to this sort of talk, it means that you're spending time with people who do yoga. And the main reason yoga practitioners talk about yoga is that they've discovered something that makes them feel good, and they want to share it with those they care about. Sorry about that. In future, we'll just let you carry on moaning about your debilitating stress, bad back and stiff shoulders, without suggesting you try the thing that cured us of exactly those things. But there is also another, wonderfully simple solution that you can implement straight away: if you don't like yogis, don't hang out with yogis. I promise, none of us will stalk you randomly to tell you about our pigeon pose. You're safe.

As for the pseudo-spiritual stuff, which is, justifiably, a

point of contention for most of the yoga bashers (and presumably what Naomi means by "vague and variable mysticism"): I don't like it either. But it doesn't have to be pseudo, and it doesn't have to be spiritual. Everything you do is what you make of it, so make of it what you like. Yoga teachers will not generally try to force the more spiritual or religious elements of the practice on you; they may be introduced as part of a class but, frankly, if you don't want to visualise the divine light entering through your third eye, or open up your heart *chakra*, there ain't a thing anyone can do about it. And if it so happens that you come across a teacher who does try to force it on you, or who puts more emphasis on the spiritual side of yoga than you like, you have a choice: go to another class. There's no shortage of options. Or stay, and take out of it what suits you, leaving the rest aside. You can do that, you know. Let's consider that excellent word, once again: *choice*. It's yours to make. Make it. Stop whining.

I won't comment on the feet; I honestly have no idea what Naomi is talking about. I have been exposed to the odd flash of genitalia, on occasions when an inappropriately tailored pair of shorts has been combined with a particularly enthusiastic one-legged dog, but I assure you, I have fully recovered. And it only took ten sessions of hypnotherapy and energy healing. But it does make me think, in cases like this, that there might be something to be said for the MC Hammer pants that Naomi accuses us of wearing.

Which brings me, neatly, to the topic of yoga attire. *Floppy*? Really? Clearly Naomi has never heard of lululemon. I am not offering this as any sort of defence;

there are many words to describe what people wear to yoga class and few of them are polite, but "floppy" is definitely not one of them. And that's all I have to say on the subject.

Let's be honest: yoga bashing is just as boring as yoga preaching, and, unless you're a priest, you can't even pretend you're doing it for the sake of our souls. And it's not just a harmless bit of fun, either. It peddles in stereotypes and preconceptions, and reinforces a narrow-minded, intolerant approach towards things that are a little unfamiliar. And it puts people off from doing yoga. For all the wrong reasons. The consensus among the yoga bashers and the yoga sceptics was that Naomi's article and the comments made in response confirmed their suspicions about yoga and put paid to any inclination they may have had to try it. One even went as far as saying he was now revising his good opinion of the friend who recommended yoga to him.

Seriously? You're gonna let a few words on a screen stand in for actual experience? Yoga may not be for everyone but if you're the slightest bit curious about it, the least you could do is try. Because the point is, *there is no such thing as yoga*. Each one of us experiences it in a completely unique way. There are dozens of different styles, and the classes on offer are probably in their millions. New batches of yoga teachers are produced practically every day and that means that, although it may still turn out that yoga is not your thing, there is a very good chance that there is some style-class-teacher combination that would suit you. Rejecting the possibility outright without even having tried is just silly. And saying that you don't like yoga after taking a class or two is almost like saying you're not into music because you heard a song once, and it wasn't very good.

So try it, and give it a proper chance, and draw your own conclusions. Or don't, but for reasons of your own, not because somebody else is offended by bare feet or loose clothing. Either way, please stop slagging it off in the name of blogging, or journalism or whatever you justify these missives as. Because, while we're on the topic, there is one rule to writing: write about what you know. And if you don't know, do your research. Thoroughly. *Learn.* If you do neither, and just produce a piece that spurts a few half-hearted stereotypes and arbitrarily attacks a particular group of people that you are neither a part of nor know very well, the result is not journalism or blogging, or a simple case of bad writing: it's bigotry. And it's really not such a fine line, actually. Take a moment to think about that and then, if you dare, glance down and check where you stand.

In closing, I would like to share some good news with those who thought sticking your head up your own arse was a skill only available to yogis, on account of our bendiness. In physical terms, this is indeed very hard to achieve, and I don't know of any yoga *asana* that prepares the body for such a feat. Take heart, however: this contortion is in fact a metaphysical one and that means that anyone can do it, without ever setting one foot in a yoga class.

Oh look – you're doing it already.

***

The title of this piece is a tribute to Tommy Ramone, the last surviving member of the punk-rock band The Ramones, who died this week. And was not a yogi, as far as I know. R.I.P. Tommy.

do you do natural yoga?

au naturel (French)
adjective & adverb
1. with no elaborate treatment, dressing or preparation
2. naked

I've spent the past two weeks on the Greek island of Sifnos, and I've been practicing yoga almost daily. Or so I thought.

Lucy, a friend of my uncle and aunt's who's spending the week here on Sifnos with us, wanted to keep up her yoga practice during her holiday. She is staying in a small and quaint complex of studio rooms overlooking the bay of Vathy. We're talking whitewashed little houses with blue shutters, and potted geraniums and basil plants dotted about a vine-shaded patio with a view of a deep, sparkling bay, and sunsets. Not a bad spot for a bit of yoga.

So Lucy sought out the landlady and asked whether there was a yoga mat she could borrow. She detected a hint of suspicion as the landlady confirmed that yes, she did have something that might work (an exercise mat, as it turned out) and went off to fetch it. When she returned, she seemed reluctant to hand it over.

'Tell me,' she enquired, 'do you plan to do your yoga in your room or out on the patio?'

'I'm not sure,' Lucy replied. 'Does it matter?'

The landlady hesitated. 'Well,' she said, 'do you do *natural* yoga?'

Lucy, naturally, struggled to answer that question

did she? She asked for some clarification.

A few years back, the landlady explained, she had a group of Swedish tourists staying, two families. They asked permission to practice yoga on the patio, and the landlady agreed. During their first session, the landlady's son, a boy of about six, came running up to her, breathless.

'Mummy!' he said. 'The ladies have black between their legs!'

Mystified, the landlady followed the boy to the patio where, true enough, in the beautiful soft light of dusk, the ladies had black between their legs, on account of performing their warriors stark naked. The landlady promptly instructed her guests that this was not the way things were done here, only to be told, amidst polite apologies and pulling on of bikinis, that they practiced *natural yoga*.

'I see,' Lucy said, when the tale came to an end. She assured the landlady that the yoga she did was by no means natural; the mat was handed over, and the appropriately clothed Lucy was able to enjoy her sun salutations without causing any children undue trauma.

As for my own practice, it takes place in my humble Sifnos yard, with a view of the mountains, and I'm usually dressed in whichever items of clothing I have to hand. Though I packed a pair of lycra shorts, two vests and a sports bra, more often than not these are either entirely forsaken or randomly combined with bikini tops, soiled t-shirts and a pair of cotton leopard print shorts that I wear to bed. I don't know if it's natural, but it's certainly *au naturel*. It's entirely free of elaborate treatment, dressing or preparation; I just throw my mat on the ground, face the mountains, and do my sun salutations.

But what is it that I'm doing, exactly?

According to my grandmother, *not* yoga. She makes this pronouncement one evening, when she spots my strap rolled up next to my mat.

'What do you use that for?' she asks disapprovingly.

'Yoga,' I reply.

'Nonsense. There are no gadgets in yoga,' she asserts. 'What would you do with it?'

'It helps me stretch my legs. Do you want to see?'

'No.' She waves her arm dismissively. 'That's not yoga. I never used any gadgets when I did yoga.'

'There are many types of yoga,' I reply, as evenly as possibly. 'Iyengar yoga uses a lot of props, actually.'

'I don't know what this Yenga might be,' she says firmly. 'But what you're doing is not yoga.'

I breathe deeply and count to ten. I don't argue.

My grandmother is only one member of the audience that my sessions seem to draw; arguably the most opinionated one. But I'm also often observed by our elderly, half-deaf neighbour – a permanent resident of the island – and her fifty year old son. Their garden offers an uninterrupted view of my mat, and they have front row seats.

'What is the girl doing?' she screeches.

'I don't know, mother,' the son bellows in response.

'She's doing yoga,' my mum supplies

'WHAT?'

'Yo-gah, mother. She says yo-gah!'

'*Ogre?*' the old woman cries desperately.

70

'YO-GAH!'

The neighbour shakes her head in irritation. 'I don't understand these things,' she mutters.

'She's doing her EXERCISE!' provides my mum, appeasingly.

'Ah, exercise. That's good. Keeping in shape. Me, I'm broken.' And she proceeds to list all of the ailments currently plaguing her.

It's very peaceful, this non-yoga of mine.

My grandmother has relented, however. Tentatively, she approached me this afternoon.

'Show me,' she ordered.

'What?'

'That nonsense you do with the strap.'

I promised I would, tonight.

She's waiting for me now. She's brought her chair out, she's got a fresh cup of coffee and some biscuits, and she's put her paper aside. She's ready to observe. So I'm going to put my laptop away, and throw on whichever top I've left hanging on the hook in the bathroom, and roll my mat out, and do whatever it is that I do every evening, as the sun sets over the mountains. I don't know what you'd call it. I don't know if it's natural or if it's even yoga. It might well be nonsense. But I like it.

the art of not practising yoga

Susanne and I had big plans for our perfect holiday. We had been looking forward to it for months: nine whole August days on a beautiful, serene Greek island; for Susanne, a sorely needed break after a year of endings, beginnings, transitions and challenges, and for me my official holiday from a gruelling, self-imposed daily writing schedule that I've followed (with varying degrees of success) since May. We would eat, drink, and explore. We would go swimming every day. We would climb a mountain. Susanne would go running; she had packed her trainers especially. And we would do yoga. Like, *all the time.*

So there we were, on Susanne's first day in Sifnos. Back at home, after a day on the beach, our faces glowing and our skin tingling from sun and sea. On the patio that I'd touted as the perfect location for outdoor yoga, with a view of monastery-topped mountains on one side, and quaint, blue-domed church on the other. The sun had begun its descent, throwing pinks and purples across the sky, as late afternoon changed into early evening. Yoga time.

And then, as I stepped over a drystone wall that I've negotiated with total success for the past twenty-odd years of my life, my foot slipped and I was sent hurtling down into a three-metre deep pit of jagged rocks, thorns and, quite possibly, snakes. Spared from breaking both my legs by virtue of some very fast reflexes and the heroic soleus muscle of my left calf, which performed some crazy ninja move and singlehandedly prevented my untimely demise. I lifted myself up and over the wall, and staggered over to where Susanne was sitting, in open-mouthed shock. We surveyed my injuries: two relatively deep, bleeding gashes on my right knee and left ankle, some superficial scrapes on my elbows, and a slight ache in my left calf. We cleaned the wounds and smothered them in coconut oil (my panacea), spent a good few minutes laughing hysterically as we both replayed the scene of me disappearing behind a wall from our respective viewpoints, and then I declared myself ready for yoga, and off I went to fetch our mats. The fact that I couldn't actually walk I attributed to shock, and dismissed: nothing was getting in the way of the first of many wonderful yoga sessions with my friend. *We had a plan.*

'I am well,' I told myself, and the Universe, and obstinately held on to this view up until the point where I tried to step back into downward dog, and my ninja soleus finally asserted itself, and I collapsed in a twisted heap in a most ungraceful manner, groaning in pain and bleeding all over my mat.

'Perhaps you could do some seated postures,' Susanne suggested, gently.

Nope. I could not.

'Maybe you should just lie down?'

This, as was established after some very awkward manoeuvring, was just about possible. So I lay on my mat, petulantly repeating 'But I want to do yoga!', while Susanne went through her practice, with frequent, nervous glances in my direction, and the sun disappeared behind the mountains.

'It'll be fine by tomorrow,' I declared confidently, as

my leg began to swell up.

It's funny, the things we take for granted. Like walking. Like getting out of bed. Like sitting on the toilet. Day two, after a sleepless night, because there was no position in which my leg didn't hurt, and it was blatantly not fine. I adopted my most cheerful disposition, regardless, winced good-naturedly whenever I moved, and tried to make plans with Susanne for going to the beach.

'I feel a bit funny,' she confessed, as – with perfect timing – a small army of builders arrived to change all the windows and doors in the house. I made Susanne coffee, of which she managed one sip before taking herself back to bed, and quickly manifested all the symptoms of moderate to acute sunstroke. So she spent the day in bed, sporting a temperature high enough to match the August heatwave (both in the 40s) and a delirious smile, while a large Georgian man drilled into the window frame barely a metre from where she lay, my mum, my grandma and my grandma's carer took turns to place compresses of cold water and vinegar on her forehead and armpits, and I lurched about the house uselessly like a comedy monster, screaming in pain at regular intervals and assuring everyone, cheerfully, that it'd all be fine by tomorrow.

Susanne did not go running; her trainers never made it out of her suitcase. And we did not climb any mountains. We went from home to beach at my slow, hobbling pace, wearing unsolicited hats (donated by family and friends who were intimately involved in Susanne's aftercare) and smothered in sun cream. We sat mostly in the shade, with Susanne allowed brief, controlled exposure to the sun and me being frequently reminded to keep my leg

74

elevated. We didn't really swim: we placed ourselves in the water and paddled about, chatting, until we got bored or cold or hungry, and made our way back to our sun loungers. On one such occasion, I balanced myself on my arms in the shallow water where the waves break, and straightened my legs back behind me, and announced to Susanne, enthusiastically: 'Look! I'm doing plank!'

Susanne shaded her eyes from the sun and regarded me critically, torn between kindness and honesty.

'No you're not,' she said finally. 'You're floating.

I had to concede this point, and the larger point at stake: I would not be doing yoga for a while. The best I could hope for was floating, and a few moments' reprieve from the pain in my leg. And that would have to be good enough.

We did no yoga, but we did eat and drink; we ate figs and almonds picked from the trees in our garden, and drank lots of iced coffee. One night, we were invited to dinner at our neighbours' house, and Eleni, our hostess, told us the tale of her first and only yoga class, and of why she hasn't tried it since. It happened in London, in the eighties, and Eleni was invited to join a friend for a one-off class, taught by a visiting guru from India. They turned up at a flat somewhere in central London, and settled down on their mats. The teacher walked in, arranged himself in lotus, and invited his students to: "Inhale. Exhale. Inhale. Exhale." His clipped Indian vowels, however, meant that the instructions that reached Eleni's ears, much like a case of broken telephone, were: "In hell. Ex hell. In hell. Ex hell." Over and over again. Convinced that she was being asked to enter and exit hell with her every breath, and that this was a necessary part of the practice, Eleni diligently spent the entire hour doing just that, and attracting some very curious glances from the teacher. By the end of the class, she was understandably both deeply distressed and exhausted by her repeated journeys in and out of hell, and quite certain that this was not an experience she'd like to repeat. Susanne and I laughed, and did nothing to try and change her mind, resisting, for once, the temptation felt by most regular yogis to convert the non-practitioners. Eleni has lived her entire life without yoga, and she is fine. She is good enough exactly as she is.

Muscle strain and sunstroke aside, or maybe because of them, Susanne and I had our perfect holiday, after all. We did no yoga, but we did explore. We explored the places we can go, the different paths we can take when unexpected limits are imposed and the usual avenues are closed. We learned to make new plans in the place of the old, and not to be too rigid about our habits – even the good ones. We learned that yoga is not for everyone and that for some it's literally hell. And we began to understand that there is an art to not practising yoga, and it's just as hard to master as its opposite. Susanne and I both struggled with it, for reasons both shared and separate, but we came through and found that it wasn't so bad. Because when something's become an established part of your life, you no longer have to fight for it; you can afford to let go of it a little, sometimes, and know that it'll still be there when you're ready to come back. And perhaps practising and not practising yoga aren't actually opposites, but parts of a much larger practice called living your life. One where muscle strain and sunstroke and aborted plans are not disasters, but things to laugh about.

Where lots of wonderful things, many of them unplanned and unexpected, take place when we step outside of the confines of our normal routines, and not doing yoga for a few days means more time spent with your friend, floating around loose-limbed in the surf under the midday sun, chatting about nothing of any consequence, and not minding your alignment one little bit.

glossary

Surya Namaskar A: Sun Salutation A
Tadasana: Mountain Pose
Urdhva Hastasana: Upward Salute
Uttanasana: Standing Forward Bend
Ardha Uttanasana: Half Standing Forward Bend
Kumbhakasana: Plank
Chaturanga Dandasana: Four-Limbed Staff Pose
Urdhva Mukha Svanasana: Upward Facing Dog
Adho Mukha Svanasana: Downward Facing Dog
Savasana: Corpse Pose; the relaxation pose generally adopted at the end of a yoga practice
Asana(s): the physical postures practiced in yoga
Pranayama: yogic techniques and exercises for regulating the breath
Ashram: a spiritual hermitage or monastery; the secluded residence of a religious community and its guru
Mudra: a symbolic hand gesture in Hinduism and Buddhism
Bandha: a Sanskrit word meaning lock, seal or bind; in yoga, an interior body "lock"
Karma yoga: the discipline of selfless action or selfless service
Satsang: a spiritual discourse or sacred gathering
Chidakasha: the psychic space in front of the closed eyes, just behind the forehead
Sankalpa: resolve, will, purpose or determination; setting an intention – crudely put, the yogic version of a New Year's resolution, but expressed in the present tense
Namaste: literally, "I bow to you"; a respectful form of greeting, acknowledgment, welcome or farewell, with the palms pressed together in front of the heart and the head slightly bowed, with or without speaking the word

Virabhadrasana II: Warrior II pose

Ujai (or *ujjayi*): a diaphragmatic breathing technique (*pranayama*) employed in various yoga practices

Dharma: (in Hinduism and Buddhism) the principles or laws that order the universe; conformity with these principles or laws

Yoga Sutras: one of the classical texts of yoga, the *Yoga Sutras* are a collection of aphorisms, compiled by Patanjali around 400 CE, that constitute the foundational text of Ashtanga Yoga

Hatha Yoga Pradipika: a classical text describing Hatha Yoga, written in the 15th century CE

Thank you for reading this little book.

If you have enjoyed it, please take a moment to rate it or post a short review on Amazon. Reviews are the single most effective way to help independent authors get more exposure, and we are always extremely grateful for them.

And tell your friends.

And maybe check out my other books on Amazon.

Do it for the pelvis!

Other things you can do from here:

Keep in touch by
joining my mailing list
for polite and infrequent
updates, news and special offers.
(No spam. Never ever.)

You might also like to sign up for
my Advance Readers' Team
and get all my new books for free
before they're released.

Or send me an email through my website:
www.daphnekapsali.com

gratitude

In May 2014, I took my life apart in order to put it back together in a way that made more sense, and be who I was truly supposed to be, full-time. It was insane; it was terrifying; it was exhilarating; it was a huge relief. It was the best thing I ever did, and I still can't believe it's worked out. But it did, and it does, and it will keep working out because that's how it goes when you start doing what's right for you. Whatever that might be.

But this has not been a solitary journey. I was helped along – sometimes nudged, sometimes carried – by a great number of amazing, kind, generous people, who have taken the time to read my work and support all of my crazy schemes, and kept me going through those inevitable moments of *what the fuck am I doing?*

All of you who bought and read my books, who shared my posts, who wrote reviews and ranted to your friends, who took the time to get in touch and tell me what the books meant to you, and your own stories. Friends and strangers, and strangers who have become friends. There are too many of you to name, but I hope you know who you are, and how grateful I am to you. Thank you all.

And thank you, once again, to my Nerd Twin, who makes me feel like less of a nerd. Except when he actually calls me a nerd.

about the author

Daphne Kapsali is a writer, reluctant yogi, pathological optimist and dedicated coffee drinker - among many other things. In 2014, she gave up her life in London to spend the autumn and winter writing on a remote Greek island called Sifnos; the result, a book entitled *100 days of solitude* – 100 separate and interconnected stories on claiming the time and space to live as your true self and do what you love – was published in March 2015 and has become an unexpected bestseller. She has since published another seven books, all of which are available from Amazon.

Daphne is a big fan of the law of attraction, the universe and all things positive, and hopes her story will keep inspiring others to overcome their fears and limiting beliefs, and live their best lives.

She and her multiple personalities divide their time between London and Sifnos, where they argue good-naturedly about who is more qualified to run their life. They have yet to reach a conclusion.

Connect:

Website: daphnekapsali.com/writing
Blog: 100daysofsolitude.com
Facebook: facebook.com/daphnewrites/
Twitter: @dafiniduck

also by daphne kapsali

100 days of solitude

you can't name an unfinished thing

collected: essays and stories on life, death and donkeys

Common People

Divided Kingdom: How Brexit made me an immigrant

Death by any other name

For Now: Notes on living a deliberate life

All my books are available to buy on Amazon, in paperback and on Kindle, or read for free on Kindle Unlimited.

Printed in Great Britain
by Amazon

49932524R00051